# The Complete Keto Diet For Beginner

Wayne Foster

ISBN: 9798698042259

# Contents

# ACKNOWLEDGMENTS

The ketogenic diet is a very low-carb, high-fat diet that shares many similarities with the Atkins and low-carb diets. It involves drastically reducing carbohydrate intake and replacing it with fat. This reduction in carbs puts your body into a metabolic state called ketosis.

When this happens, your body becomes incredibly efficient at burning fat for energy. It also turns fat into ketones in the liver, which can supply energy for the brain (Trusted Source, Trusted Source). Ketogenic diets can cause massive reductions in blood sugar and insulin levels. This, along with the increased ketones, has numerous health benefits

# 1.WHAT IS A KETO DIET?

A keto diet is well known for being a low carb diet, where the body produces ketones in the liver to be used as energy. It's referred to as many different names – ketogenic diet, low carb diet, low carb high fat (LCHF), etc.

When you eat something high in carbs, your body will produce glucose and insulin.

Glucose is the easiest molecule for your body to convert and use as energy so that it will be chosen over any other energy source.

Insulin is produced to process the glucose in your bloodstream by taking it around the body.

Since the glucose is being used as a primary energy, your fats are not needed and are therefore stored. Typically on a normal, higher carbohydrate diet, the body will use glucose as the main form of energy. By lowering the intake of carbs, the body is induced into a state known as ketosis.

Ketosis is a natural process the body initiates to help us survive when food intake is low. During this state, we produce ketones, which are produced from the breakdown of fats in the liver.

The end goal of a properly maintained keto diet is to force your body into this metabolic state. We don't do this through starvation of calories but starvation of carbohydrates.

## What Do I Eat on a Keto Diet?

To start a keto diet, you will want to plan ahead. That means having a viable diet plan ready and waiting. What you eat depends on how fast you want to get into a ketogenic state (ketosis). The more restrictive you are on your carbohydrates (less than 25g net carbs per day), the faster you will enter ketosis.

You want to keep your carbohydrates limited, coming mostly from vegetables, nuts, and dairy. Don't eat any refined carbohydrates such as wheat (bread, pasta, cereals), starch (potatoes, beans, legumes) or fruit. The small exceptions to this are avocado, star fruit, and berries which can be consumed in moderation.

*Do Not Eat*

- Grains – wheat, corn, rice, cereal, etc.

- Sugar – honey, agave, maple syrup, etc.

- Fruit – apples, bananas, oranges, etc.

- Tubers – potato, yams, etc.

*Do Eat*

- Meats – fish, beef, lamb, poultry, eggs, etc.

- Leafy Greens – spinach, kale, etc.

- Above ground vegetables – broccoli, cauliflower, etc.

- High Fat Dairy – hard cheeses, high fat cream, butter, etc.

- Nuts and seeds – macadamias, walnuts, sunflower seeds, etc.

- Avocado and berries – raspberries, blackberries, and other low glycemic impact berries

- Sweeteners – stevia, erythritol, monk fruit, and other low-carb sweeteners >

- Other fats – coconut oil, high-fat salad dressing, saturated fats, etc.

To see more specific advice on what (and what not) to eat, see our full keto food list >

Try to remember that keto is high in fat, moderate in protein, and very low in carbs. Your nutrient intake should be something around 70% fats, 25% protein, and 5% carbohydrate.

Typically, anywhere between 20-30g of net carbs is recommended for everyday dieting – but the lower you keep your carbohydrate intake and glucose levels, the better the overall results will be. If you're doing keto for weight loss, it's a good idea to keep track of both your total carbs and net carbs.

Protein should always be consumed as needed with fat filling in the remainder of the calories in your day.

You might be asking, "What's a net carb?" It's simple really! The net carbs are your total dietary carbohydrates, minus the total fiber. I recommend keeping total carbs below 35g and net carbs below 25g (ideally, below 20g).

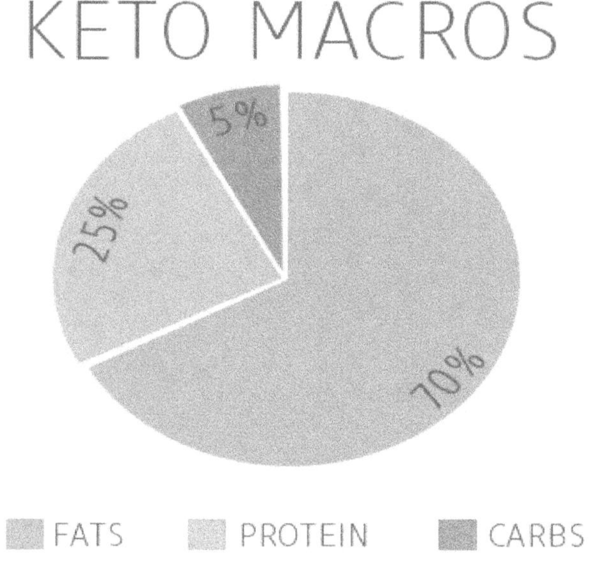



If you're finding yourself hungry throughout the day, you can snack on nuts, seeds, cheeses, or almond butter to curb your appetite (though snacking can slow progress in the long term). Sometimes we can confuse the want to snack with the need for a meal. If you're in a rush and need a keto fast food option, there are some available.

**Vegetables on a Ketogenic Diet**

Dark green and leafy is always the best choice for vegetables. Most of your meals should be a protein with vegetables, and an extra side of fat. Chicken thighs basted in olive oil, with broccoli and cheese. Steak topped with a knob of butter, and a side of spinach sauteed in olive oil.

If you're still confused about what a net carb is, don't worry – I'll explain further. Let's say for example you want to eat some broccoli (1 cup) – one of my favorite keto vegetables out there.

- There are a total of 6g carbohydrates in 1 cup.

- There's also 2g of fiber in 1 cup.

- So, we take the 6g (*total carbs*) and subtract the 2g (*dietary fiber*).

- This will give us our net carbs of 4g.

Here's a list of the most common low carb vegetables. Though if you want a complete list, check out our guide on the best vegetables for a

ketogenic diet

| Vegetable | Amount | Net Carbs |
| --- | --- | --- |
| Spinach (Raw) | 1/2 Cup | 0.1 |
| Bok Choi (Raw) | 1/2 Cup | 0.2 |
| Lettuce (Romaine) | 1/2 Cup | 0.2 |
| Cauliflower (Steamed) | 1/2 Cup | 0.9 |
| Cabbage (Green Raw) | 1/2 Cup | 1.1 |
| Cauliflower (Raw) | 1/2 Cup | 1.4 |
| Broccoli (Florets) | 1/2 Cup | 2 |
| Collard Greens | 1/2 Cup | 2 |
| Kale (Steamed) | 1/2 Cup | 2.1 |
| Green Beans (Steamed) | 1/2 Cup | 2.9 |

# 2. BENEFITS OF A KETO DIET

There is a ton of hype surrounding the ketogenic diet. Some researchers swear that it is the best diet for most people to be on, while others think it is just another fad diet.

To some degree, both sides of the spectrum are right. There isn't one perfect diet for everyone or every condition, regardless of how many people "believe" in it. The ketogenic diet is no exception to this rule.

However, the ketogenic diet also has plenty of solid research backing up its benefits. In fact, it has been found to be better than most diets at helping people with:

- Epilepsy
- Type 2 Diabetes
- Type 1 Diabetes
- High Blood Pressure
- Alzheimer's disease
- Parkinson's disease
- Chronic Inflammation
- High Blood Sugar Levels

- Obesity
- Heart Disease
- Polycystic Ovary Syndrome
- Fatty Liver Disease
- Cancer
- Migraines

Even if you are not at risk from any of these conditions, the ketogenic diet can be helpful for you too. Some of the benefits that most people experience are:

- Better brain function
- A decrease in inflammation
- An increase in energy
- Improved body composition

As you can see, the ketogenic diet has a wide array of benefits, but is it any better than other diets?

**The Calorie Conundrum**

Many researchers argue that ketosis (burning ketones for fuel) and carbohydrate restrictions only play a minor role in the benefits of the ketogenic diet. Their argument is that people tend to eat fewer calories on the ketogenic diet, and this is the main reason for its benefits.

It is true that people on the ketogenic diet tend to eat less because of how satiating eating a high-fat moderate-protein diet is for us. And it is also true that less calorie consumption leads to improved health and weight loss, but there is something that many researchers don't consider.

The ketogenic diet elicits many other important mechanisms in the body and cells that are nonexistent in other diets. These unique mechanisms explain the benefits of the ketogenic diet that eating fewer calories cannot.

**How The Body Adapts To The Ketogenic Diet — The Main Reason for Many of the Benefits**

*From The Cell's Point of View*

Carbohydrates are the body's preferred fuel source. When its consumption is restricted, the body reacts as if it is fasting. This stimulates new energy pathways to provide energy for the cells. One of these energy pathways is called ketogenesis, and the result of ketogenesis is an alternative fuel source called a ketone body.

These ketones bodies can be used by almost every cell in your body for fuel (except for the liver and red blood cells). However, sugar and ketone bodies affect the body in many different ways.

For example, burning sugar for fuel creates more reactive oxygen species. These reactive oxygen species cause damage, inflammation, and cell death when they accumulate. This is why consuming too much sugar is known to impair brain function and cause plaque build up in the brain.

On the other hand, ketones provide a more efficient energy source and help protect neuron cells in the brain. This is partly because burning ketones for fuel decreases the production of reactive oxygen species and enhances mitochondrial function and production.

The healthy cells that are struggling to survive are helped by the carbohydrate restriction as well. Without access to carbohydrates, a cellular process called autophagy is activated. This process up-regulates many factors that improve cell health and resilience, clean up the cell from damage and elicit anti-inflammatory processes.

The combination of autophagy and ketone burning are essential in helping people with cancer and brain disorders like epilepsy, migraines, and Alzheimer's.

*From The Body's Perspective*

Now, let's zoom out and look at how the ketogenic diet changes the body. It all begins with a change in insulin levels.

By restricting carbohydrates, we take the biggest stimulator of insulin out of the diet. This decreases insulin levels, increases fat burning, and reduces inflammation. The combination of these three changes addresses the primary drivers of many chronic diseases — insulin resistance, inflammation, and fat accumulation.

*The Takeaway — The Mechanisms Behind The Ketogenic Diet*

From a mechanistic level, here is why the ketogenic diets can lead to benefits that reach beyond caloric restriction:

On a cellular level:

- Ketones burn more efficiently than sugar.
- Carbohydrate restriction triggers autophagy and anti-inflammatory processes.
- Burning ketones for fuel creates less reactive oxygen species.
- Ketone usage enhances mitochondrial function and production.

In the body:

- Insulin levels decrease because dietary carbohydrate isn't stimulating its release.
- Fat burning increases because the body needs to use alternative fuel sources.
- Inflammation is reduced because inflammatory fat levels decrease and less reactive oxygen species are formed.

The combination of the cellular and bodily effects of the ketogenic diet provides us with a basis for why they may be useful in the treatment of the conditions we mentioned earlier. However, this is only biochemistry. Is the ketogenic diet scientifically proven to help people with those conditions?

*Treating Epilepsy — The Origins of The Ketogenic Diet*

Our journey through the research on the ketogenic diet starts in 1924 with Dr. Russell Wilder. At the prestigious Mayo Clinic, Dr. Wilder designed a carbohydrate-restricted diet to treat epilepsy in children, and the research at the time indicated that it was highly effective.

The first high-quality study on epilepsy and the ketogenic diet wasn't published until much later, in 1998. In this study, researchers recruited 150 children, and nearly all of them had more than two seizures per week despite taking at least two seizure-reducing medications. The children were provided with a ketogenic diet for a one-year trial.

After three months, about 34% of the children, or slightly over one-third, had over a 90% decrease in seizures.

Keto originated to help treat epilepsy in children.

After six months, 71% of the children remained on the ketogenic diet, and about 32% had over a 90% reduction in seizures. After a full year, 55% stayed on the diet and 27% at least a 90% decrease in seizures.

Thus, the researchers stated that the ketogenic diet is "more effective than many of the new anticonvulsant medications and is well tolerated by children and families when it is effective." Not only was the ketogenic diet helpful, but it was more helpful than some commonly used drugs.

More recently, a meta-analysis was published in the Journal of Neurology that assessed the impact of the ketogenic diet in treating epilepsy. It included a total of 19 studies with a total of 1084 patients. After analyzing the data, the researchers noted that the patients who stayed on the diet had a 2.25 times greater probability of treatment success (at least a 50% reduction in seizures).

The Takeaway: With or without the help of medication, the ketogenic diet is effective in reducing seizures.

Recommendations: If conventional therapies are not helping you or your child lower the frequency of seizures, strongly consider using a ketogenic diet. Remember to discuss a suitable plan with your doctor and a registered dietitian, and monitor its effectiveness. Use Ruled.me to gain access to critical information on the keto lifestyle and community that will help you stick to the diet.

**The Ketogenic Diet in Reversing Type 2 Diabetes**

Insulin resistance is a widespread problem that, if not properly managed, can lead to prediabetes and eventually type 2 diabetes. Thankfully, abundant research suggests that modifying your diet to a low-carbohydrate or ketogenic diet can help people lower their insulin to healthy levels and reverse insulin resistance.

In fact, after analyzing the data from 10 randomized trials on using diet to treat diabetes, researchers found that a low-carbohydrate diet has a greater effect on blood sugar control in type 2 diabetics than high-carbohydrate diets.

They even found a distinct relationship between carbohydrate restriction and blood sugar lowering. Less carbohydrate consumption meant better blood sugar levels.

Research shows that a ketogenic diet can help reverse type 2 diabetes.

It's that simple — put people with prediabetes or type 2 diabetes on a low-carbohydrate ketogenic diet, and their health improves, blood sugar levels drop, and insulin sensitivity increases. Even studies that put healthy individuals on a ketogenic diet found similar improvements.

The Takeaway: The ketogenic diet is highly effective at reversing type 2 diabetes.

Recommendations: If you have type 2 diabetes or any blood sugar issues, consider implementing the

**How to Lower Your Blood Sugar Naturally**

Controlling Type 1 Diabetes with the Ketogenic Diet

Type 1 diabetes causes the same blood sugar control issues as type 2 diabetes, but in an entirely different way. Type 1 diabetics cannot produce enough insulin or any insulin at all, which requires them to have insulin administered exogenously. On top of that, the perfect diet will not be able to reverse this disease as the ketogenic diet can for type 2 diabetes.

However, there may be a perfect diet to help manage type 1 diabetes.

One case report of a 19-year-old male with Type 1 diabetes found that a paleolithic ketogenic diet may have the ability "to halt or reverse autoimmune processes destructing pancreatic beta cell function in [Type 1

Diabetes].” In other words, a ketogenic diet consisting of low-carbohydrate whole-foods may be able to reverse type 1 diabetes!

Keto can help control blood sugars for Type 1 diabetics.

Although it is a stretch to say that a paleolithic ketogenic diet can reverse type 1 diabetes, a recent critical evaluation of the literature confirms that the ketogenic diet is the best-documented diet for controlling type 1 diabetes.

The group of 26 leading researchers stated that there is

“…evidence supporting the use of low-carbohydrate diets as the first approach to treating type 2 diabetes and as the most effective adjunct to pharmacology in type 1. They represent the best-documented, least controversial results.”

The Takeaway: A whole-food-based ketogenic diet is the best diet for keeping type 1 diabetes under control and may even help treat it.

Recommendations: if you have type 1 diabetes, a whole-food based ketogenic diet may be the best diet for you. However, make sure you consult with your doctor about adjusting your treatment plan before making these changes.

Improving Blood Pressure With the Ketogenic Diet

A ketogenic diet can improve blood pressure.

According to the World Health Organization, high blood pressure is estimated to cause about 12.8% of the total of all deaths. Luckily, The ketogenic diet may be the solution, according to a 2007 study.

In this study, researchers compared the impact of a low-carbohydrate diet and three other diets on blood pressure and other measures of cardiovascular fitness in women. After the 12 month trial, all subjects who successfully completed their respective diet experienced notable reductions in body mass, triglycerides, and LDL cholesterol. Those in the low-carbohydrate diet group, however, had the best results.

These participants decreased their systolic blood pressure by an average of 7.6 mm Hg — twice more than any other group. Their diastolic pressure also decreased by 2.93% from 75 mm Hg to 72.8 mm Hg.

These findings were confirmed in another interesting study. Researchers compared the effects of the low-carbohydrate diet to the effects of a combination of a low-fat diet and orlistat (a weight-loss and blood pressure lowering medication) on blood pressure. The researchers stated that the low-carbohydrate dietary intervention "was more effective for lowering blood pressure."

Does this mean that you should throw away your blood pressure medication and dive into the ketogenic diet? Not just yet — you should first consult with your dietitian or doctor to see if cutting some carbs is a suitable strategy for you

The Takeaway: A low-carbohydrate diet is more effective than a low-fat and moderate-fat diet at reducing blood pressure. Limiting carbohydrates even produces better results than the combination of a low-fat diet and a weight-loss/blood pressure drug.

Recommendations: If you are interested in lowering blood pressure, a diet with 50 or fewer grams of carbohydrates per day might be an effective method. Consult with your doctor and dietitian to see if it's a suitable choice based on your medical history.

**The Power to Improve the Alzheimer's Disease**

The ketogenic diet has the power to improve Alzheimer's disease symptoms.

Earlier in this article, I briefly mentioned how consuming too much sugar can impair brain function and cause plaque build up in the brain. Many studies on Alzheimer's disease patients agree with the biochemistry as well. In fact, A group of scientists reviewed the literature and concluded that "high carbohydrate intake worsens cognitive performance and behavior in patients with Alzheimer's disease." This means that eating more carbohydrates cause more problems in the brain. Will the opposite (eating fewer carbs) improve brain function?

Recent studies on the ketogenic diet provide evidence that it may be able to reverse Alzheimer's disease. Experiments on ketone supplementation specifically found that the ketone body,  β-hydroxybutyrate, improved memory function of Alzheimer's patients.

Scientists validated this finding by giving MCT oil (a fat found in coconut oil that is usually converted into ketones in the liver) to Alzheimer's patients and tested their memory. They found that the Alzheimer's patients experienced greater memory recall that directly correlated with their blood levels of ketone bodies.

Other benefits that ketone bodies have on brain health are:

They prevent neuronal loss.

They preserve neuron function.

They protect brain cells against multiple types of injury.

The Takeaway: The combination of carbohydrate restriction and ketones improves brain function and may help prevent and reverse Alzheimer's disease. Conversely, a high-carbohydrate diet is deleterious to brain health.

Recommendations: Try supplementing with MCT oil and restricting carbohydrates to improve brain function and prevent (or reduce the severity of) Alzheimer's disease.

**Parkinson's Disease Symptoms Reduced By Ketogenic Diet**

One recently published clinical study tested the effects of the ketogenic diet on symptoms of Parkinson's disease. In this study, Parkinson's disease patients experienced a mean of 43% reduction in Unified Parkinson's Disease Rating Scale scores after a 28-day ketogenic diet.

All participating patients reported moderate to very good improvement in symptoms. The researchers hypothesize that these results are partly due to the increase in essential fatty acid consumption that is common with ketogenic diets.

The Takeaway: The ketogenic diet improves the quality of life and reduces the symptoms of patients with Parkinson's disease.

Recommendations: If you have or are developing  Parkinson's disease, speak to your doctor about going on a ketogenic diet and join the Ruled.me community for support.

## Improve Cholesterol Levels and Reverse Heart Disease with The Ketogenic Diet

A ketogenic diet can help improve cholesterol levels.

Although the ketogenic diet tends to be high in saturated fat (commonly thought to increase cholesterol), it has been found to improve cholesterol levels and reduce the risk of heart disease.

In a recent meta-analysis published in the British Journal of Nutrition, researchers investigated the impacts of very-low-carbohydrate ketogenic diets (VLCKD) on key metrics of cardiovascular health including HDL cholesterol. The authors defined a VLCKD as a diet of less than 50g of carbohydrates.

After examining 12 studies including 1257 patients, they found that the VLCKD increases HDL by double the average increase in HDL of the low-fat dieters. As a result, the authors concluded that carbohydrate-restricted diets confer cardiovascular benefits because they improve levels on HDL in the body.

However, one of the most important risk factors for heart disease is the "bad" LDL cholesterol. How does the ketogenic impact LDL cholesterol levels?

In a 2006 study, researchers assessed the effects of carbohydrate restriction on LDL cholesterol in a group of 29 men for a 12-week weight-loss intervention. Their LDL cholesterol levels improved, leading to the conclusion that:

…weight loss induced by carb restriction favorably alters the secretion and processing of plasma lipoproteins, rendering VLDL, LDL, and HDL particles associated with decreased risk for atherosclerosis and coronary heart disease.

In another study on women, researchers confirmed that the ketogenic diet resulted in favorable changes in LDL particles consistent with lower cardiovascular disease risk. However, the total LDL cholesterol did not change. This is why it is important to test the levels of different LDL particles. Looking at the LDL number itself may be misleading, especially on the ketogenic diet.

The Takeaway: Low carbohydrate diets can help optimize cholesterol levels, and reduce the risk of heart disease.

Recommendations: If you have high levels of LDL particles and VLDL particles, consider adopting a carbohydrate-restricted diet. To optimize your LDL cholesterol levels, consider adopting a diet high in healthy monounsaturated fats and low-carb vegetables. Some examples of keto-friendly foods that are high in monounsaturated fats are olive oil, avocado, and macadamia nuts.

**A Potential Treatment for Polycystic Ovary Syndrome and Infertility**

Polycystic ovary syndrome (PCOS) is responsible for as much as 70 percent of infertility issues in women.

The primary cause of this condition is elevated insulin levels. When insulin levels are high, they cause the ovaries to produce more androgens (like testosterone) and decrease the production of sex-hormone binding globulin — a glycoprotein that prevents testosterone from freely entering cells.

With more androgen production and less sex-hormone binding globulin, free testosterone can freely float through the blood and interact with cells. Depending on what cells it influences, this can result in hair growth on the chest and face, mood swings, fatigue, low sex drive, acne, infertility and other PCOS symptoms.

A ketogenic diet can help reduce or even reverse the symptoms of PCOS.

As androgen levels continue to increase, they stimulate 5-alpha reductase activity — an enzyme that converts testosterone to a more potent metabolite called dihydrotestosterone. This makes PCOS symptoms even worse.

The research on how diet affects PCOS is minimal, but there is one compelling study on the ketogenic diet and women with PCOS. In this study, five overweight women ate a ketogenic diet (20 grams of carbohydrates or less per day) for 24 weeks. The results were astounding — average weight loss was 12%, free testosterone decreased by 22%, and fasting insulin levels dropped by 54%. What's even more impressive is that two of the women became pregnant despite previous infertility problems.

Although this is a small study, the results are clearly backed by the fact that the ketogenic diet has been found in many other studies to help reverse insulin resistance and reduce insulin levels, the two main causes of PCOS.

The Takeaway: The ketogenic diet can help improve fertility and reverse PCOS.

Recommendations: If you have PCOS, then carbohydrate restriction may work for you. However, there is one important caveat for women who are on the ketogenic diet. The diet may increase cortisol levels, which results in increased insulin resistance. For some women, it may be best to reduce carbohydrate intake slowly.

### Reverse Non-Alcoholic Fatty Liver Disease with the Ketogenic Diet

A ketogenic diet can help with non alcoholic fatty liver disease.

Non-alcoholic fatty liver disease is associated with type 2 diabetes, obesity, heart disease, and hyperlipidemia, and it probably will not develop unless one or more of these issues are present as well.

We've already explored how the ketogenic diet helps with diabetes, heart disease, and hyperlipidemia, does this mean it helps with non-alcoholic fatty liver disease as well?

A recent pilot study put five patients on the ketogenic diet (less than 20 grams per day of carbohydrate). At the end of six months, the average weight loss was 28 pounds (but this wasn't the most surprising finding). Each patient underwent a liver biopsy, and four of the five patients had a reduction in liver fat, inflammation, and fibrosis. However, this is a small pilot study that also used supplements, so the results are not conclusive. What does the rest of the research say?

In a 2016 meta-analysis and systematic review, the researchers found that the low carbohydrate diet decreased fat in the liver significantly, but liver function tests did not improve significantly. When we look closely at the studies in the meta-analysis, they either found no effect on liver enzyme levels or a significant effect. In other words, the liver function of some people stayed the same on the low-carbohydrate diet while others improved significantly. Why the difference?

My guess is that if subjects were required to eat more fibrous foods (like low-carbohydrate vegetables), then they probably would have had results similar to the small pilot study.

The Takeaway: A whole food based ketogenic diet may be the best diet for reversing fatty liver disease.

Recommendations: If you have fatty liver disease, then start restricting carbohydrates and eating low-carb vegetables like spinach, kale, and broccoli with every meal.

## The Ketogenic Diet Helps Cancer Patients

Recently, there has been more talk about the potential of ketogenic diet being a cancer treatment, but what does the available literature have to say about that?

A recent meta-analysis looked at the literature on 32 glioma patients (people that had a tumor in their brain or spinal cord) treated using the ketogenic diet as an alternative or complementary therapy. The researchers noted that some patients were more responsive to the ketogenic diet than other patients were.

The best response was in a 3-year-old girl who had complete remission after five years of treatment with a ketogenic diet. Two other patients also experienced complete remission after the diet, while another experienced cancer progression after stopping the diet.

Keto can help fight cancer.

These are incredible results, but we must remember that these results are due to a combination of a ketogenic diet and conventional treatment, not the ketogenic diet alone.

It is evident, however, that the ketogenic diet is one of the best diets for cancer patients. According to dietitian Heidi H. Pfeifer at the MGH Center for Dietary Therapy, the ketogenic diet may be effective because of the following two reasons.

First, the ketogenic diet deprives cancer cells of their primary source of energy — glucose. While many of the cancer cells are starving, the body is running on ketones, which the cancer cells cannot use for fuel.

Second, the ketogenic diet suppresses insulin like growth factor (IGF-1). This molecule is associated with the formation and progression of cancerous cells. IGF-1 levels are increased when we eat more carbohydrates. Because the ketogenic diet is much lower in carbohydrates, scientists suspect that this suppresses IGF-1 production, slowing the formation of cancerous cells.

The Takeaway: The ketogenic diet is one of the best complementary treatments for people who have cancer.

Recommendations: Ask your doctor about including the ketogenic diet in your cancer treatment program, and use Ruled.me for support and guidance through your recovery process.

**Prevent and Reduce the Severity of Migraines**

A ketogenic diet has been shown to reduce the severity of migraines.

The first study on the Ketogenic diet and how it affects migraines came a few years after its first use for epilepsy in 1928. The study was done on 28 patients, and only 9 of them showed  "some improvement" although most of them admitted poor compliance.

In a review of the research on the ketogenic diet and migraines (over seventy years later), the scientists  concluded that the ketogenic diet "ameliorates headaches and reduces drug consumption in migraineurs, while the SD [standard low-calorie diet] is fully ineffective on migraine in a short term observation."

The researchers hypothesized that the positive effects that the ketogenic diet has on migraines are due to how ketone bodies inhibit neural inflammation and enhance brain mitochondrial metabolism. The ketone bodies do this by blocking high concentrations of glutamate (commonly found in both migraine and epilepsy sufferers) and reducing oxidative stress.

The Takeaway: The ketogenic diet and ketones are an effective treatment for migraineurs.

Recommendations: If you suffer from migraines or recurring headaches, consider trying the ketogenic diet to get into ketosis or taking supplemental ketones in the form of MCT oil. Combining MCT oil with the ketogenic diet will probably give you the best results.

# 3. FULL KETO DIET FOOD LIST

Eat

Here are the foods that you can eat on a ketogenic diet:

### Meat

Meat – Unprocessed meats are low carb and keto-friendly, and organic and grass-fed meat might be even healthier.1 But remember that keto is a higher-fat diet, not high in protein, so you don't need huge amounts of meat. Excess protein (over 2.0 g per kg of reference body weight; see this chart to determine your own protein targets) can be converted to glucose, which could make it harder for some people to get into ketosis, especially when starting out and with high levels of insulin resistance

### Fish and seafood

These are all good, especially fatty fish like salmon. If you have concerns about mercury or other toxins, consider eating more of the smaller fish like sardines, mackerel and herring. If you can find wild-caught fish, that's probably the best. Avoid breading, as it contains carbs

### Eggs

Eat them any way you want, e.g. boiled, fried in butter, scrambled or as omelets.

Buying organic or pastured eggs might be the healthiest option, although we do not have scientific studies to prove better health.4How many eggs can you eat, considering cholesterol? Our advice is no more than 36 eggs, per day.5 But feel free to eat fewer if you prefer.

### Fats&sauces

Natural fat, high-fat sauces – Most of the calories on a keto diet should come from fat. You'll likely get much of it from natural sources like meat, fish, eggs, and other sources. But also use fat in cooking, like butter or coconut oil, and feel free to add plenty of olive oil to salads and vegetables. You can also eat delicious high-fat sauces, including Bearnaise sauce, garlic butter, and others

### Keto low-carb vegetables

Vegetables growing above ground. Fresh or frozen – either is fine. Choose vegetables growing above ground (here's why), especially leafy and green items. Favorites include cauliflower, cabbage, avocado, broccoli and zucchini.

Vegetables are a tasty way to eat good fat on keto. Fry them in butter and pour plenty of olive oil on your salad. Some even think of vegetables as a fat-delivery system. They also add more variety, flavor and color to your keto meals.

Many people end up eating more vegetables than before when starting keto, as veggies replace the pasta, rice, potatoes, and other starches. It's even possible to eat a vegetarian or vegan keto diet.

### Keto dairy

High-fat dairy – Butter is good, high-fat cheese is fine, and heavy cream is great for cooking.

Avoid drinking milk as the milk sugar quickly adds up (one glass = 15 grams of carbs), but you can use it sparingly in your coffee. What does "sparingly" mean? That depends on how many cups per day you drink! We recommend one cup with just a "splash," about a tablespoon max. But even better is to do away with the milk completely.

Definitely avoid caffè latte (18 grams of carbs). Also avoid low-fat yogurts, especially as they often contain lots of added sugars.

Finally, be aware that regularly snacking on cheese when you're not hungry is a common mistake that can slow weight loss.

### Keto nuts

Nuts – Can be had in moderation, but be careful when using nuts as snacks, as it's very easy to eat far more than you need to feel satisfied. Also be aware that cashews are relatively high carb, choose macadamia or pecan nuts instead or check out our full keto nuts guide

How much is too much? That depends on your weight loss progress and the rest of your carb intake. As a general rule, try to limit nut intake to less than 1/2 cup per day (around 50 grams).

### Berries

Berries – A moderate amount is OK on keto, perhaps with real whipping cream, a popular keto dessert.

In summary, eat real low-carb foods like meat, fish, eggs, vegetables and natural fats like butter or olive oil. As a basic beginner's rule, stick to foods with fewer than 5% carbs (numbers below).

### Drink

Here is a list of what you can drink on a ketogenic diet:

Water – The #1 option. Have it flat, with ice, or sparkling. Sip it hot like a tea, or add natural flavouring like sliced cucumbers, lemons, or limes. If you experience headaches or symptoms of "keto flu", add a few shakes of salt to your water.

Coffee – No sugar. A small amount of milk or cream is fine. For extra energy from fat, stir in butter and coconut oil for "Bulletproof coffee." Note, if weight loss stalls, cut back on the cream or fat in your coffee.

Tea – Whether black, green, Orange Pekoe, mint, or herbal — feel free to drink most teas. Don't add sugar.

Bone broth – Hydrating, satisfying, full of nutrients and electrolytes — and simple to make! — homemade bone broth can be a great beverage to sip on the keto diet. Stir in a pat of butter for some extra energy

*Tips:Keto drinks – the best and the worst*

**Size mattersSize matters**

Drinking a sugary soft drink on a keto diet is never a good idea, but size truly matters. A large bottle (i.e 33 ounces or 1 liter or more) has more carbs than almost an entire week's keto allowance.

A can of soda can kick you out of ketosis for a day, but a large bottle may prevent ketosis for a number of days or even a week.

If you have diabetes or insulin resistance, avoid all sugary soft drinks in order to keep your blood glucose stable and improve your health.

**Low-Carb Diet DrinksDiet sodas — yay or nay?**

Over the last 40 years, diet sodas — without calories or carbs — have had a huge market around the world, promoting the idea that you can have a sugary-tasting beverage without any of the harms and consequences of real sugar. Alas, it is not that simple.

Sweetened with artificial products like aspartame, sucralose, acesulfame K or refined stevia, these diet drinks are not necessarily helpful for sustained weight loss or improved health.

Their problems include maintaining cravings for sweet tastes, which can undermine keto progress and keep sugar addictions in place.5 Acting on the same taste bud sensors as real sugar, they blunt the ability to taste the natural flavors and sweetness of real food. Some sweeteners, such as sucralose, can still cause a blood glucose and insulin response and contribute to fat storage. Observational studies show that drinking diet soft drinks is associated with higher BMIs and higher rates of cardiovascular disease.

Other studies have noted that their long term impact on many health factors is still unknown, but that they may alter many body processes, such as metabolism, brain reward systems, appetite regulation, and the microbiome.

Studies supporting the use of diet soft drinks in weight loss programs are often conducted by the diet drink industry. A 2017 study found that much of the research on artificial sweeteners has been funded by industry and features conflict of interest, research bias, and positive results that cannot be reproduced.

Drinking diet soda may or may not be better than drinking sugary soda. However, one thing is certain. If you can cut both out of your daily beverage habits, your health and waistline will likely thank you.

### Keto alcoholAlcohol on keto: yea or nay?

Unlike most diets, which usually forbid all alcohol, the keto diet allows moderate consumption of specific alcoholic beverages

Dry red and white wine is fine in moderation. Beer is generally not okay — it is liquid bread — but there are a few low carb beers that can be consumed from time to time. And spirits — like vodka, gin or whiskey — have no carbs at all.

### Detailed carb-count list for common drinks

Remember that a strict keto diet, keeps carbs very low. It is typically best to keep carbs from drinks as close to 0 as possible and to use your carb allotment for foods such as fresh vegetables. Below is a detailed list of the number of grams of carbs in a typical serving size of various drinks.

**Water 0** (The clear winner)
**Water with lemon 0**
**Tea 0** (one sugar cube adds 4 grams)
**Keto iced tea 0** (recipe)

**Coffee 0** (milk adds roughly 1-3 grams of carbs)
**Diet soft drink 0** (artificial sweeteners cause other problems though)
**Wine 2** (5 oz – 14 cl)
**Almond milk, unsweetened 2** (8 oz – 25 cl)
**Coconut water 9** (1 cup – 24 cl)
**Vegetable juice 11** (1 cup – 24 cl). The amount of carbs can vary. Adding fruit juice adds more carbs.
**Milk 11** (1 cup – 24 cl). Lactose, the sugar in milk can be problematic for some.
**Soy milk 12** (1 cup – 24 cl)
**Beer 13** (12 oz – 35 cl). The amount varies (keto beer guide).
**Caffè latte 15** (12 oz – 35 cl)
**Kombucha tea 10** (12 oz – 35 cl). This is the average of commercial teas. Homemade Kombucha tea varies with the time it has fermented, and may end up somewhat lower in carbs.
**Orange juice 26** (1 cup – 24 cl)
**Energy drink 28** (8.4 oz – 25 cl)
**Vitamin water 32** (12 oz – 35 cl)
**Sweetened iced tea 32** (12 oz – 35 cl). This is the average of most commercial iced tea products, which vary in their amount of sweetness.
**Soft drink 39** (12 oz – 35 cl)
**Smoothie 36** (12 oz – 35 cl). Varies depending on contents. May be low carb, but not typically keto ratios. (Low-carb smoothie recipes).
**Frappuccino 50** (12 oz – 35 cl). All sweet coffee drinks are high in carbs.
**Milkshake 60** (10 oz – 30 cl). Not part of a ketogenic diet.


**Avoid:** Aavoid on a keto diet – foods containing a lot of carbs, both the sugary and the starchy kind. This includes starchy foods like bread, pasta, rice and potatoes. These foods are very high in carbs.

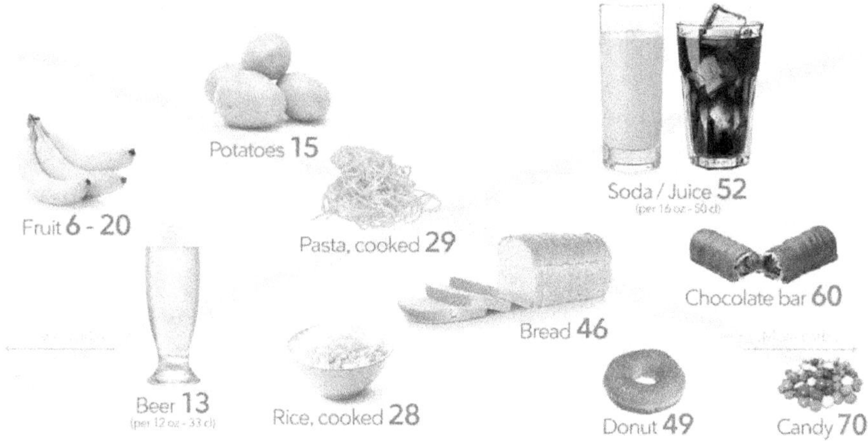


The numbers are grams of net carbs per 100 grams (3.5 ounces), unless otherwise noted.

Also avoid or limit highly processed foods and instead follow our whole foods keto diet advice.

You should also avoid low-fat diet products. A keto diet should be moderately high in protein and will probably be higher in fat, since fat provides the energy you're no longer getting from carbohydrate. Low-fat products usually provide too many carbs and not enough protein and fat.

What to drink

What can you drink on a ketogenic diet? Water is the perfect drink, and coffee or tea are fine too. Ideally, use no sweeteners, especially sugar.18

A splash of milk or cream in your coffee or tea is OK, but beware that the carbs can add up if you drink multiple cups in a day (and definitely avoid caffe lattes

## ABOUT THE AUTHOR

I am Wayne Foster. I'm a student in university. I've compiled a great list here and I've excited they're all in the one spot. I hope you enjoy it as much as I enjoyed making it!

When you finish this book it would be amazing if you could leave a review for me as it'd mean the world.

Thanks so much for reading by my little corner.

Hope you enjoy the book

www.ingramcontent.com/pod-product-compliance
Lightning Source LLC
Chambersburg PA
CBHW052137150726
48002CB00006B/2655